This Playbook Belongs To Coach:

_____

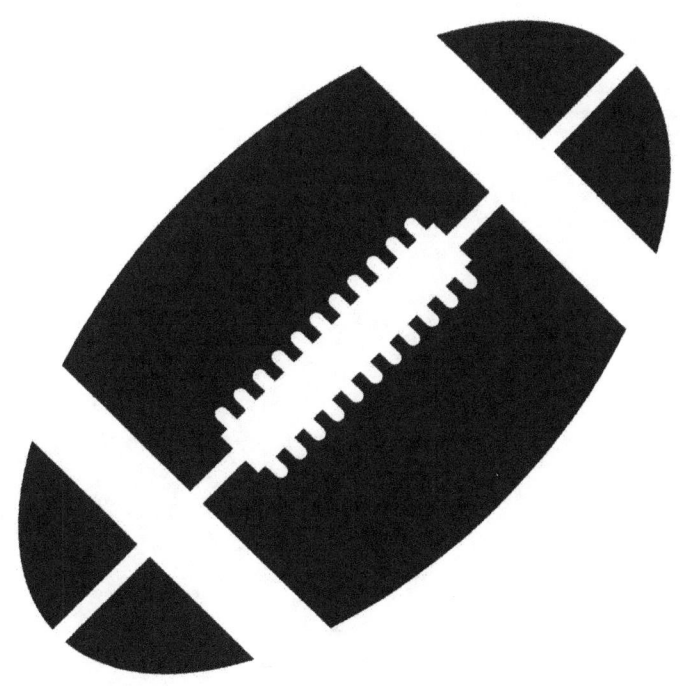

DEDICATION

This Football Coach Playbook is dedicated to all the coaches out there who want to keep track of their plays and game stats, and document their findings in the process.

You are my inspiration for producing books and I'm honored to be a part of keeping all of your Football notes and records organized.

This journal notebook will help you record your details about tracking your plays and game statistics.

Thoughtfully put together with these sections to record: 12 Monthly Undated Calendar Month Pages, 20 Blank Football Field Templates, 20 Game Statistics Pages, and Notes.

HOW TO USE THIS BOOK

The purpose of this book is to keep all of your Football notes all in one place. It will help keep you organized.

This Football Coach Playbook will allow you to accurately document every detail about your coaching.

Here are examples of the prompts for you to fill in and write about your experience in this book:

1. 12 Monthly Undated Calendar Month Pages - Write down practices, camps, special training, an overview of games that month, or anything else you want to log.

2. 20 Blank Football Field Templates - Write out your plays.

3. 20 Game Statistics Pages - Record date, opponent, teams scores for each quarter, players name, tackles, assists, total sacks, QB sacks, fumbles, and much more.

4. Notes - Plenty of notes pages to write any additional important information such as thoughts about games, different tactics that are working or needed work, tasks, drills, or anything else you're planning for your team.

Month Of

SUN	MON	TUES	WED	THURS	FRI	SAT

Month Of

SUN	MON	TUES	WED	THURS	FRI	SAT

Month Of

SUN	MON	TUES	WED	THURS	FRI	SAT

Month Of

SUN	MON	TUES	WED	THURS	FRI	SAT

Month Of

SUN	MON	TUES	WED	THURS	FRI	SAT

Month Of

SUN	MON	TUES	WED	THURS	FRI	SAT

Month Of

SUN	MON	TUES	WED	THURS	FRI	SAT

Month Of

SUN	MON	TUES	WED	THURS	FRI	SAT

Month Of

SUN	MON	TUES	WED	THURS	FRI	SAT

Month Of

SUN	MON	TUES	WED	THURS	FRI	SAT

Month Of

SUN	MON	TUES	WED	THURS	FRI	SAT

Month Of

SUN	MON	TUES	WED	THURS	FRI	SAT

Game Statistics

Game Date:_____   Opponent: _____   H/A

Score

	1ST QTR	2ND QTR	3RD QTR	FINAL
US				
OPPONENT				

PLAYER	SOLO TACKLES	ASSISTS	TOTAL SACKS	QB SACKS	TACKLE LOSS	INT	FUMBLES CAUSED	FUMBLE RECOV.

PLAYER	SOLO TACKLES	ASSISTS	TOTAL SACKS	QB SACKS	TACKLE LOSS	INT	FUMBLES CAUSED	FUMBLE RECOV.
PLAYER	SOLO TACKLES	ASSISTS	TOTAL SACKS	QB SACKS	TACKLE LOSS	INT	FUMBLES CAUSED	FUMBLE RECOV.

Game Statistics

Game Date:_____   Opponent: _____   H/A

Score

	1ST QTR	2ND QTR	3RD QTR	FINAL
US				
OPPONENT				

PLAYER	SOLO TACKLES	ASSISTS	TOTAL SACKS	QB SACKS	TACKLE LOSS	INT	FUMBLES CAUSED	FUMBLE RECOV.

PLAYER	SOLO TACKLES	ASSISTS	TOTAL SACKS	QB SACKS	TACKLE LOSS	INT	FUMBLES CAUSED	FUMBLE RECOV.
PLAYER	SOLO TACKLES	ASSISTS	TOTAL SACKS	QB SACKS	TACKLE LOSS	INT	FUMBLES CAUSED	FUMBLE RECOV.

Game Statistics

Game Date:_____   Opponent: _____   H/A

Score

	1ST QTR	2ND QTR	3RD QTR	FINAL
US				
OPPONENT				

PLAYER	SOLO TACKLES	ASSISTS	TOTAL SACKS	QB SACKS	TACKLE LOSS	INT	FUMBLES CAUSED	FUMBLE RECOV.

PLAYER	SOLO TACKLES	ASSISTS	TOTAL SACKS	QB SACKS	TACKLE LOSS	INT	FUMBLES CAUSED	FUMBLE RECOV.
PLAYER	SOLO TACKLES	ASSISTS	TOTAL SACKS	QB SACKS	TACKLE LOSS	INT	FUMBLES CAUSED	FUMBLE RECOV.

Game Statistics

Game Date: _____   Opponent: _____   H/A

Score

	1ST QTR	2ND QTR	3RD QTR	FINAL
US				
OPPONENT				

PLAYER	SOLO TACKLES	ASSISTS	TOTAL SACKS	QB SACKS	TACKLE LOSS	INT	FUMBLES CAUSED	FUMBLE RECOV.

PLAYER	SOLO TACKLES	ASSISTS	TOTAL SACKS	QB SACKS	TACKLE LOSS	INT	FUMBLES CAUSED	FUMBLE RECOV.
PLAYER	SOLO TACKLES	ASSISTS	TOTAL SACKS	QB SACKS	TACKLE LOSS	INT	FUMBLES CAUSED	FUMBLE RECOV.

Game Statistics

Game Date:_____   Opponent: _____   H/A

Score

	1ST QTR	2ND QTR	3RD QTR	FINAL
US				
OPPONENT				

PLAYER	SOLO TACKLES	ASSISTS	TOTAL SACKS	QB SACKS	TACKLE LOSS	INT	FUMBLES CAUSED	FUMBLE RECOV.

PLAYER	SOLO TACKLES	ASSISTS	TOTAL SACKS	QB SACKS	TACKLE LOSS	INT	FUMBLES CAUSED	FUMBLE RECOV.
PLAYER	SOLO TACKLES	ASSISTS	TOTAL SACKS	QB SACKS	TACKLE LOSS	INT	FUMBLES CAUSED	FUMBLE RECOV.

Game Statistics

Game Date: _____   Opponent: _____   H/A

Score

	1ST QTR	2ND QTR	3RD QTR	FINAL
US				
OPPONENT				

PLAYER	SOLO TACKLES	ASSISTS	TOTAL SACKS	QB SACKS	TACKLE LOSS	INT	FUMBLES CAUSED	FUMBLE RECOV.

PLAYER	SOLO TACKLES	ASSISTS	TOTAL SACKS	QB SACKS	TACKLE LOSS	INT	FUMBLES CAUSED	FUMBLE RECOV.
PLAYER	SOLO TACKLES	ASSISTS	TOTAL SACKS	QB SACKS	TACKLE LOSS	INT	FUMBLES CAUSED	FUMBLE RECOV.

Game Statistics

Game Date:_____ Opponent: _____ H/A

Score

	1ST QTR	2ND QTR	3RD QTR	FINAL
US				
OPPONENT				

PLAYER	SOLO TACKLES	ASSISTS	TOTAL SACKS	QB SACKS	TACKLE LOSS	INT	FUMBLES CAUSED	FUMBLE RECOV.

PLAYER	SOLO TACKLES	ASSISTS	TOTAL SACKS	QB SACKS	TACKLE LOSS	INT	FUMBLES CAUSED	FUMBLE RECOV.
PLAYER	SOLO TACKLES	ASSISTS	TOTAL SACKS	QB SACKS	TACKLE LOSS	INT	FUMBLES CAUSED	FUMBLE RECOV.

Game Statistics

Game Date: _____   Opponent: _____   H/A

Score

	1ST QTR	2ND QTR	3RD QTR	FINAL
US				
OPPONENT				

PLAYER	SOLO TACKLES	ASSISTS	TOTAL SACKS	QB SACKS	TACKLE LOSS	INT	FUMBLES CAUSED	FUMBLE RECOV.

PLAYER	SOLO TACKLES	ASSISTS	TOTAL SACKS	QB SACKS	TACKLE LOSS	INT	FUMBLES CAUSED	FUMBLE RECOV.
PLAYER	SOLO TACKLES	ASSISTS	TOTAL SACKS	QB SACKS	TACKLE LOSS	INT	FUMBLES CAUSED	FUMBLE RECOV.

Game Statistics

Game Date:_____   Opponent: _____   H/A

Score

	1ST QTR	2ND QTR	3RD QTR	FINAL
US				
OPPONENT				

PLAYER	SOLO TACKLES	ASSISTS	TOTAL SACKS	QB SACKS	TACKLE LOSS	INT	FUMBLES CAUSED	FUMBLE RECOV.

PLAYER	SOLO TACKLES	ASSISTS	TOTAL SACKS	QB SACKS	TACKLE LOSS	INT	FUMBLES CAUSED	FUMBLE RECOV.
PLAYER	SOLO TACKLES	ASSISTS	TOTAL SACKS	QB SACKS	TACKLE LOSS	INT	FUMBLES CAUSED	FUMBLE RECOV.

Game Statistics

Game Date: _____   Opponent: _____   H/A

Score

	1ST QTR	2ND QTR	3RD QTR	FINAL
US				
OPPONENT				

PLAYER	SOLO TACKLES	ASSISTS	TOTAL SACKS	QB SACKS	TACKLE LOSS	INT	FUMBLES CAUSED	FUMBLE RECOV.

PLAYER	SOLO TACKLES	ASSISTS	TOTAL SACKS	QB SACKS	TACKLE LOSS	INT	FUMBLES CAUSED	FUMBLE RECOV.
PLAYER	SOLO TACKLES	ASSISTS	TOTAL SACKS	QB SACKS	TACKLE LOSS	INT	FUMBLES CAUSED	FUMBLE RECOV.

Game Statistics

Game Date:_____ Opponent: _____ H/A

Score

	1ST QTR	2ND QTR	3RD QTR	FINAL
US				
OPPONENT				

PLAYER	SOLO TACKLES	ASSISTS	TOTAL SACKS	QB SACKS	TACKLE LOSS	INT	FUMBLES CAUSED	FUMBLE RECOV.

PLAYER	SOLO TACKLES	ASSISTS	TOTAL SACKS	QB SACKS	TACKLE LOSS	INT	FUMBLES CAUSED	FUMBLE RECOV.
PLAYER	SOLO TACKLES	ASSISTS	TOTAL SACKS	QB SACKS	TACKLE LOSS	INT	FUMBLES CAUSED	FUMBLE RECOV.

Game Statistics

Game Date:_____   Opponent: _____   H/A

Score

	1ST QTR	2ND QTR	3RD QTR	FINAL
US				
OPPONENT				

PLAYER	SOLO TACKLES	ASSISTS	TOTAL SACKS	QB SACKS	TACKLE LOSS	INT	FUMBLES CAUSED	FUMBLE RECOV.

PLAYER	SOLO TACKLES	ASSISTS	TOTAL SACKS	QB SACKS	TACKLE LOSS	INT	FUMBLES CAUSED	FUMBLE RECOV.
PLAYER	SOLO TACKLES	ASSISTS	TOTAL SACKS	QB SACKS	TACKLE LOSS	INT	FUMBLES CAUSED	FUMBLE RECOV.

Game Statistics

Game Date: _____   Opponent: _____   H/A

Score

	1ST QTR	2ND QTR	3RD QTR	FINAL
US				
OPPONENT				

PLAYER	SOLO TACKLES	ASSISTS	TOTAL SACKS	QB SACKS	TACKLE LOSS	INT	FUMBLES CAUSED	FUMBLE RECOV.

PLAYER	SOLO TACKLES	ASSISTS	TOTAL SACKS	QB SACKS	TACKLE LOSS	INT	FUMBLES CAUSED	FUMBLE RECOV.
PLAYER	SOLO TACKLES	ASSISTS	TOTAL SACKS	QB SACKS	TACKLE LOSS	INT	FUMBLES CAUSED	FUMBLE RECOV.

Game Statistics

Game Date: _____   Opponent: _____   H/A

Score

	1ST QTR	2ND QTR	3RD QTR	FINAL
US				
OPPONENT				

PLAYER	SOLO TACKLES	ASSISTS	TOTAL SACKS	QB SACKS	TACKLE LOSS	INT	FUMBLES CAUSED	FUMBLE RECOV.

PLAYER	SOLO TACKLES	ASSISTS	TOTAL SACKS	QB SACKS	TACKLE LOSS	INT	FUMBLES CAUSED	FUMBLE RECOV.
PLAYER	SOLO TACKLES	ASSISTS	TOTAL SACKS	QB SACKS	TACKLE LOSS	INT	FUMBLES CAUSED	FUMBLE RECOV.

Game Statistics

Game Date: _____   Opponent: _____   H/A

Score

	1ST QTR	2ND QTR	3RD QTR	FINAL
US				
OPPONENT				

PLAYER	SOLO TACKLES	ASSISTS	TOTAL SACKS	QB SACKS	TACKLE LOSS	INT	FUMBLES CAUSED	FUMBLE RECOV.

PLAYER	SOLO TACKLES	ASSISTS	TOTAL SACKS	QB SACKS	TACKLE LOSS	INT	FUMBLES CAUSED	FUMBLE RECOV.
PLAYER	SOLO TACKLES	ASSISTS	TOTAL SACKS	QB SACKS	TACKLE LOSS	INT	FUMBLES CAUSED	FUMBLE RECOV.

Game Statistics

Game Date:_____   Opponent: _____   H/A

Score

	1ST QTR	2ND QTR	3RD QTR	FINAL
US				
OPPONENT				

PLAYER	SOLO TACKLES	ASSISTS	TOTAL SACKS	QB SACKS	TACKLE LOSS	INT	FUMBLES CAUSED	FUMBLE RECOV.

PLAYER	SOLO TACKLES	ASSISTS	TOTAL SACKS	QB SACKS	TACKLE LOSS	INT	FUMBLES CAUSED	FUMBLE RECOV.
PLAYER	SOLO TACKLES	ASSISTS	TOTAL SACKS	QB SACKS	TACKLE LOSS	INT	FUMBLES CAUSED	FUMBLE RECOV.

Game Statistics

Game Date: _____   Opponent: _____   H/A

Score

	1ST QTR	2ND QTR	3RD QTR	FINAL
US				
OPPONENT				

PLAYER	SOLO TACKLES	ASSISTS	TOTAL SACKS	QB SACKS	TACKLE LOSS	INT	FUMBLES CAUSED	FUMBLE RECOV.

PLAYER	SOLO TACKLES	ASSISTS	TOTAL SACKS	QB SACKS	TACKLE LOSS	INT	FUMBLES CAUSED	FUMBLE RECOV.
PLAYER	SOLO TACKLES	ASSISTS	TOTAL SACKS	QB SACKS	TACKLE LOSS	INT	FUMBLES CAUSED	FUMBLE RECOV.

Game Statistics

Game Date:_____   Opponent: _____   H/A

Score

	1ST QTR	2ND QTR	3RD QTR	FINAL
US				
OPPONENT				

PLAYER	SOLO TACKLES	ASSISTS	TOTAL SACKS	QB SACKS	TACKLE LOSS	INT	FUMBLES CAUSED	FUMBLE RECOV.

PLAYER	SOLO TACKLES	ASSISTS	TOTAL SACKS	QB SACKS	TACKLE LOSS	INT	FUMBLES CAUSED	FUMBLE RECOV.
PLAYER	SOLO TACKLES	ASSISTS	TOTAL SACKS	QB SACKS	TACKLE LOSS	INT	FUMBLES CAUSED	FUMBLE RECOV.

Game Statistics

Game Date:_____   Opponent: _____   H/A

Score

	1ST QTR	2ND QTR	3RD QTR	FINAL
US				
OPPONENT				

PLAYER	SOLO TACKLES	ASSISTS	TOTAL SACKS	QB SACKS	TACKLE LOSS	INT	FUMBLES CAUSED	FUMBLE RECOV.

PLAYER	SOLO TACKLES	ASSISTS	TOTAL SACKS	QB SACKS	TACKLE LOSS	INT	FUMBLES CAUSED	FUMBLE RECOV.
PLAYER	SOLO TACKLES	ASSISTS	TOTAL SACKS	QB SACKS	TACKLE LOSS	INT	FUMBLES CAUSED	FUMBLE RECOV.

Game Statistics

Game Date: _____   Opponent: _____   H/A

Score

	1ST QTR	2ND QTR	3RD QTR	FINAL
US				
OPPONENT				

PLAYER	SOLO TACKLES	ASSISTS	TOTAL SACKS	QB SACKS	TACKLE LOSS	INT	FUMBLES CAUSED	FUMBLE RECOV.

PLAYER	SOLO TACKLES	ASSISTS	TOTAL SACKS	QB SACKS	TACKLE LOSS	INT	FUMBLES CAUSED	FUMBLE RECOV.
PLAYER	SOLO TACKLES	ASSISTS	TOTAL SACKS	QB SACKS	TACKLE LOSS	INT	FUMBLES CAUSED	FUMBLE RECOV.

Notes

Notes

Notes

Notes

Notes

Notes

Notes

Notes

Notes

Notes

Notes

Notes

Notes

Notes

Notes

Notes

Notes

Notes

Notes

Notes

Notes

Notes

Notes

Notes

Notes

Notes

Notes

Notes

Notes

Notes

Notes

Notes

Notes

Notes

Notes

Notes

Notes

www.ingramcontent.com/pod-product-compliance
Lightning Source LLC
Chambersburg PA
CBHW081231080526
44587CB00022B/3897